Amazing Keto Chaffle for everyone

50 quick and good recipes easy to prepare

Catherine Willis

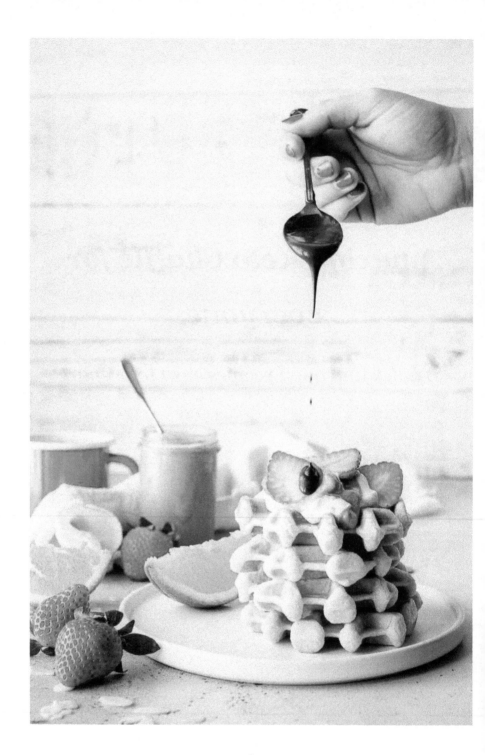

sources. Please consult a licensed professional before attempting any techniques outlined in this book.

By reading this document, the reader agrees that under no circumstances is the author responsible for any losses, direct or indirect, which are incurred as a result of the use of information contained within this document, including, but not limited to, — errors, omissions, or inaccuracies.

Table of Contents

Butter & Cream Cheese Chaffles

Preparation time : 8 minutes

Cooking Time : 16 Minutes

Servings : 2

INGREDIENTS :

> 2 tablespoons butter, melted and cooled
>
> 2 large organic eggs
>
> 2 ounces cream cheese, softened
>
> ¼ cup powdered erythritol
>
> 1½ teaspoons organic vanilla extract
>
> Pinch of salt
>
> ¼ cup almond flour
>
> 2 tablespoons coconut flour
>
> 1 teaspoon organic baking powder

DIRECTIONS :

1. Preheat a mini waffle iron and then grease it.
2. In a bowl, add the butter and eggs and beat until creamy.
3. Add the cream cheese, erythritol, vanilla extract, and salt, and beat until well combined.

4. Add the flours and baking powder and beat until well combined.
5. Place ¼ of the mixture into preheated waffle iron and cook for about 4 minutes.
6. Repeat with the remaining mixture.
7. Serve warm.

NUTRITION :

Calories 217 Net Carbs 3.3 g Total Fat 1g Saturated Fat 8.8 gCholesterol 124 mgSodium 173 mg Total Carbs 6.6 gFiber 3.3 g Sugar 1.2 gProtein 5.3 g

Cinnamon Chaffles

Preparation time : 5 minutes

Cooking Time : 8 Minutes

Servings : 2

INGREDIENTS :

　　1 large organic egg, beaten

　　¾ cup mozzarella cheese, shredded

　　½ tablespoon unsalted butter, melted

　　2 tablespoons blanched almond flour

　　2 tablespoons erythritol

½ teaspoon ground cinnamon

　　½ teaspoon Psyllium husk powder

　　¼ teaspoon organic baking powder

　　½ teaspoon organic vanilla extract

　　Topping

　　1 teaspoon powdered Erythritol

　　¾ teaspoon ground cinnamon

DIRECTIONS :

1. Preheat a waffle iron and then grease it.
2. For chaffles: In a medium bowl, put all ingredients and with a fork, mix until well combined.

9

3. Put a portion of the mixture into preheated waffle iron and cook for about 5 minutes.

4. Repeat with the remaining mixture.

5. Meanwhile, for topping: in a small bowl, mix the erythritol and cinnamon.

6. Place the chaffles onto serving plates and set aside to cool slightly.

7. Sprinkle with the cinnamon mixture and serve immediately.

NUTRITION :

Calories 142 Net Carbs 2.1 g Total Fat 10.6 g Saturated Fat 4 gCholesterol 106 mgSodium 122 mg Total Carbs 4.1 gFiber 2 g Sugar 0.3 gProtein 7.7 g

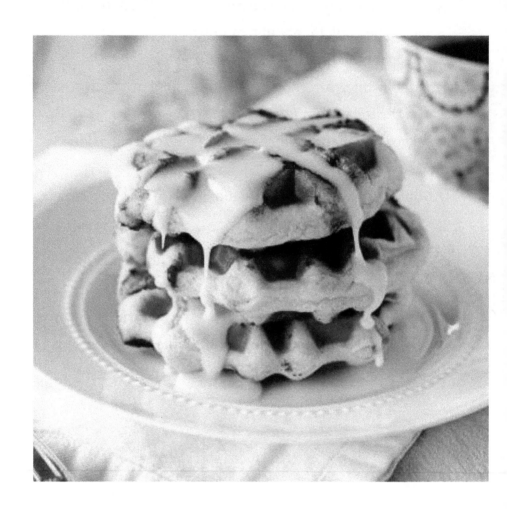

Glazed Chaffles

Preparation time : 5 minutes

Cooking Time : 5 Minutes

Servings : 2

INGREDIENTS :

½ cup mozzarella shredded cheese

⅛ cup cream cheese

2 Tbsp unflavored whey protein isolate

2 Tbsp swerve confectioners' sugar substitute

½ tsp baking powder

½ tsp vanilla extract

1 egg

For the glaze topping:

2 Tbsp heavy whipping cream

3-4 Tbsp swerve confectioners' sugar substitute

½ tsp vanilla extract

DIRECTIONS :

1. Turn on the waffle maker to heat and oil it with cooking spray.

2. In a microwave-safe bowl, mix mozzarella and cream cheese. Heat at 30 second intervals until melted and fully combined.

3. Add protein, 2 Tbsp sweetener, baking powder to cheese. Knead with hands until well incorporated.

4. Place dough into a mixing bowl and beat in egg and vanilla until a smooth batter forms.

5. Put ⅓ of the batter into the waffle maker, and cook for 3-minutes, until golden brown.

6. Repeat until all 3 chaffles are made.

7. Beat glaze **INGREDIENTS** in a bowl and pour over chaffles before serving.

NUTRITION :

Carbs: 4 g;Fat: 6 g;Protein: 4 g;Calories: 130

Blueberry Cream Cheese Chaffles

Preparation time : 5 minutes

Cooking Time : 8 Minutes

Servings : 2

INGREDIENTS :

    1 organic egg, beaten

    1 tablespoon cream cheese, softened

    3 tablespoons almond flour

    ¼ teaspoon organic baking powder

    1 teaspoon organic blueberry extract

    5-6 fresh blueberries

DIRECTIONS :

1. Preheat a mini waffle iron and then grease it.
2. In a bowl, place all the ingredients except blueberries and beat until well combined.
3. Fold in the blueberries.
4. Divide the mixture into 5 portions.
5. Place 1 portion of the mixture into preheated waffle iron and cook for about 3-4 minutes or until golden brown.
6. Repeat with the remaining mixture.
7. Serve warm.

NUTRITION :

Calories: 120Net Carb: 1.Fat: 9.6gSaturated Fat: 2.2gCarbohydrates: 3.1gDietary Fiber: 1.3g Sugar: 1gProtein: 3.2g

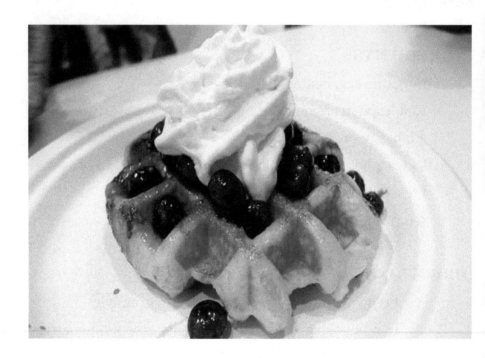

Italian Cream Waffle Sandwich-cake

Preparation time : 8 minutes

Cooking Time : 20 Minutes

INGREDIENTS :

6 oz cream cheese

4 eggs

1 Tbsp melted butter

1 tsp vanilla extract

½ tsp cinnamon

1 Tbsp monk fruit sweetener

4 Tbsp coconut flour

1 Tbsp almond flour

1½ teaspoons baking powder

1 Tbsp coconut, shredded and unsweetened

1 Tbsp walnuts, chopped

For the Italian cream frosting:

2 Tbsp butter room temp

2 Tbsp monk fruit sweetener

½ tsp vanilla

DIRECTIONS :

1. Combine cream cheese, eggs, melted butter, vanilla, sweetener, flours, and baking powder in a blender.

2. Add walnuts and coconut to the mixture.

3. Blend to get a creamy mixture.
4. Turn on the waffle maker to heat and oil it with cooking spray.
5. Add enough batter to fill the waffle maker. Cook for 2-3 minutes, until chaffles are done.
6. Remove and let them cool.
7. Mix all frosting ingredients in another bowl. Stir until smooth and creamy.
8. Frost the chaffles once they have cooled.
9. Top with cream and more nuts.

NUTRITION :

Carbs: 31 g;Fat: 2 g;Protein: 5 g;Calories: 168

Whipping Cream Chaffles

Preparation time : 5 minutes

Cooking Time : 8 Minutes

Servings : 2

INGREDIENTS :

    1 organic egg, beaten

    1 tablespoon heavy whipping cream

    2 tablespoons sugar-free peanut butter powder

    2 tablespoons Erythritol

    ¼ teaspoon organic baking powder

    ¼ teaspoon peanut butter extract

DIRECTIONS :

1. Preheat a mini waffle iron and then grease it.
2. Add all ingredients in a medium bowl and, with a fork, mix until well mixed.
3. Put half of the mixture in the preheated waffle iron and cook until golden brown, or around 4 minutes.
4. Repeat with the mixture that remains.
5. Serve it hot.

NUTRITION :

Calories: 112Net Carb: 1.Fat: 6.9gSaturated Fat: 2.7gCarbohydrates: 3.7gDietary Fiber: 2.1g Sugar: 0.2gProtein: 10.9g

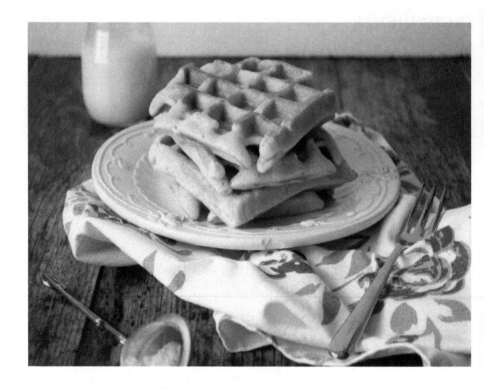

Cinnamon Pumpkin Waffles

Preparation time : 8 minutes

Cooking Time : 16 Minutes

Servings : 2

INGREDIENTS :

    2 organic eggs

    2/3 cup Mozzarella cheese, shredded

    3 tablespoons sugar-free pumpkin puree

    3 teaspoons almond flour

    2 teaspoons granulated Erythritol

    2 teaspoons ground cinnamon

DIRECTIONS :

1. Preheat a mini waffle iron and then grease it.
2. Add all ingredients in a medium bowl and, with a fork, mix until well mixed.
3. Put half of the mixture in the preheated waffle iron and cook until golden brown, or around 4 minutes.
4. Repeat with the mixture that remains.
5. Serve it hot.

NUTRITION :

Calories: Net Carb: 1.4gFat: 4gSaturated Fat: 1.3gCarbohydrates: 2.5gDietary Fiber: 1.1g Sugar: 0.6gProtein: 4.3g

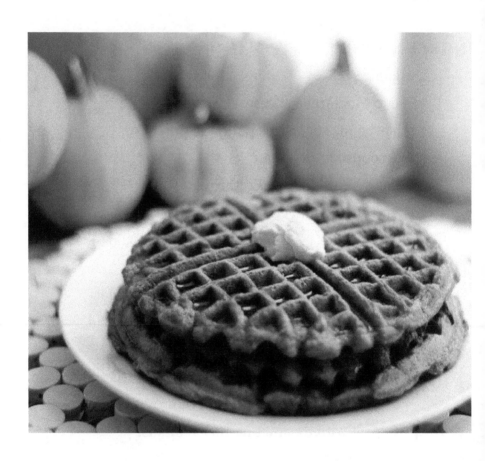

Garlic Mayo Vegan Chaffles

Servings :2

Cooking Time :5minutes

INGREDIENTS:

1 tbsp. chia seeds

2 ½ tbsps. water

¼ cup low carb vegan cheese

2 tbsps. coconut flour

1 cup low carb vegan cream cheese, softened

1 tsp. garlic powder

pinch of salt

2 tbsps. vegan garlic mayo for topping

DIRECTIONS:

1. Preheat your square waffle maker.
2. Mix chia seeds and water, let it stand for 5 minute suites.
3. Add all ingredients to the chia seeds mixture and mix well.
4. Pour vegan chaffle batter in a greased waffle maker
5. Cover and cook for about 3-minute suites.
6. Once chaffles are cooked, remove from the maker.
7. Top with garlic mayo and pepper.

8. Enjoy!

NUTRITION:

Protein: 42kcal Fat: 82kcal Carbohydrates: 6kcal

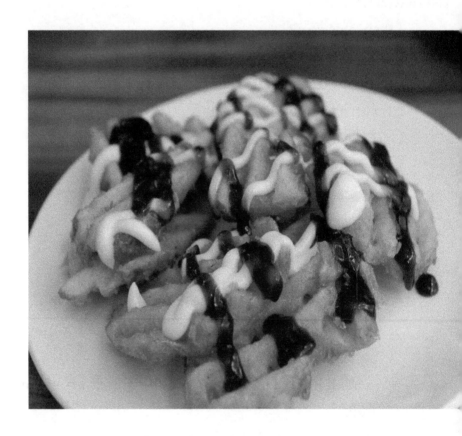

Broccoli Chaffle

Servings :4

Cooking Time :15 Minutes

INGREDIENTS:

Batter

4 eggs

2 cups grated mozzarella cheese

1 cup steamed broccoli, chopped

Salt and pepper to taste

1 clove garlic, minced

1 teaspoon chili flakes

2 tablespoons almond flour

2 teaspoons baking powder

2 tablespoons cooking spray to brush the waffle maker

¼ cup mascarpone cheese for serving

DIRECTIONS:

1. Preheat the waffle maker.
2. Add the eggs, grated mozzarella, chopped broccoli, salt and pepper, minced garlic, chili flakes, almond flour and baking powder to a bowl.
3. Mix with a fork.

4. Brush the heated waffle maker with cooking spray and add a few tablespoons of the batter.

5. Cover and cook for about 7 minutes depending on your waffle maker.

6. Serve each chaffle with mascarpone cheese.

NUTRITION:

Calories 229, fat 15 g, carbs 6 g, sugar 1.1 g,Protein 13.1 g, sodium 194 mg

Celery And Cottage Cheese Chaffle

Servings :4

Cooking Time :15 Minutes

INGREDIENTS:

Batter

4 eggs

2 cups grated cheddar cheese

1 cup fresh celery, chopped

Salt and pepper to taste

2 tablespoons chopped almonds

2 teaspoons baking powder

2 tablespoons cooking spray to brush the waffle maker

¼ cup cottage cheese for serving

DIRECTIONS:

1. Preheat the waffle maker.
2. Add the eggs, grated mozzarella cheese, chopped celery, salt and pepper, chopped almonds and baking powder to a bowl.
3. Mix with a fork.
4. Brush the heated waffle maker with cooking spray and add a few tablespoons of the batter.

5. Cover and cook for about 7 minutes depending on your waffle maker.

6. Serve each chaffle with cottage cheese on top.

NUTRITION:

Calories 385, fat 31.6 g, carbs 4 g, sugar 1.5 g,Protein 22.2 g, sodium 492 mg

Mushroom And Almond Chaffle

Servings :4

Cooking Time :15 Minutes

INGREDIENTS:

Batter

4 eggs

2 cups grated mozzarella cheese

1 cup finely chopped zucchini

3 tablespoons chopped almonds

2 teaspoons baking powder

Salt and pepper to taste

1 teaspoon dried basil

1 teaspoon chili flakes

2 tablespoons cooking spray to brush the waffle maker

DIRECTIONS:

1. Preheat the waffle maker.
2. Add the eggs, grated mozzarella, mushrooms, almonds, baking powder, salt and pepper, dried basil and chili flakes to a bowl.
3. Mix with a fork.
4. Brush the heated waffle maker with cooking spray and add a few tablespoons of the batter.

28

5. Cover and cook for about 7 minutes depending on your waffle maker.

6. Serve and enjoy.

NUTRITION:

Calories 196, fat 16 g, carbs 4 g, sugar 1 g,Protein 10.8 g, sodium 152 mg

Spinach And Artichoke Chaffle

Servings :4

Cooking Time :15 Minutes

INGREDIENTS:

Batter

4 eggs

2 cups grated provolone cheese

1 cup cooked and diced spinach

½ cup diced artichoke hearts

Salt and pepper to taste

2 tablespoons coconut flour

2 teaspoons baking powder

Other

2 tablespoons cooking spray to brush the waffle maker

¼ cup of cream cheese for serving

DIRECTIONS:

1. Preheat the waffle maker.
2. Add the eggs, grated provolone cheese, diced spinach, artichoke hearts, salt and pepper, coconut flour and baking powder to a bowl.
3. Mix with a fork.
4. Brush the heated waffle maker with cooking spray and add a few tablespoons of the batter.

5. Cover and cook for about 7 minutes depending on your waffle maker.

6. Serve each chaffle with cream cheese.

NUTRITION:

Calories 42 fat 32.8 g, carbs 9.5 g, sugar 1.1 g,Protein 25.7 g, sodium 722 mg

Avocado Croque Madame Chaffle

Servings :4

Cooking Time :15 Minutes

INGREDIENTS:

Batter

4 eggs

2 cups grated mozzarella cheese

1 avocado, mashed

Salt and pepper to taste

6 tablespoons almond flour

2 teaspoons baking powder

1 teaspoon dried dill

2 tablespoons cooking spray to brush the waffle maker

4 fried eggs

2 tablespoons freshly chopped basil

DIRECTIONS:

1. Preheat the waffle maker.
2. Add the eggs, grated mozzarella, avocado, salt and pepper, almond flour, baking powder and dried dill to a bowl.
3. Mix with a fork.

4. Brush the heated waffle maker with cooking spray and add a few tablespoons of the batter.

5. Cover and cook for about 7 minutes depending on your waffle maker.

6. Serve each chaffle with a fried egg and freshly chopped basil on top.

NUTRITION:

Calories 393, fat 32.1 g, carbs 9.2 g, sugar 1.3 g,Protein 18.8 g, sodium 245 mg

Fruity Vegan Chaffles

Servings :2

Cooking Time :5minutes

INGREDIENTS:

1 tbsp. chia seeds

2 tbsps. warm water

¼ cup low carb vegan cheese

2 tbsps. strawberry puree

2 tbsps. Greek yogurt

pinch of salt

DIRECTIONS:

1. Preheat minutesi waffle maker to medium-high heat.
2. Mix chia seeds and water and let it stand for a few minutes until it thickens.
3. Mix the rest of the ingredients in chia seed egg and mix well.
4. Spray waffle machine with cooking spray.
5. Introduce vegan waffle batter into the center of the waffle iron.
6. Cover and cook chaffles for about 3-5 minute suites.
7. Once cooked, remove from the maker and serve with berries on top.

NUTRITION:

Protein: 32% Fat: 63% Carbohydrates: 5%

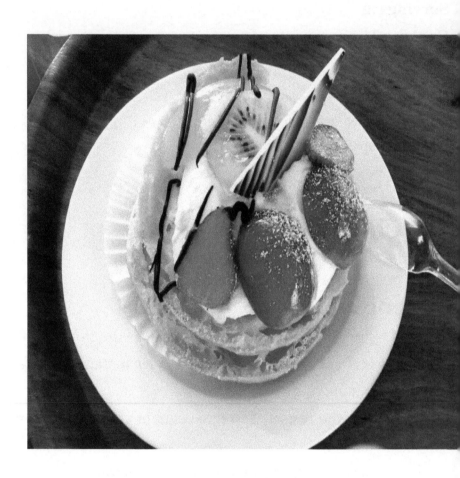

Almonds And Flax Seeds Chaffles

Servings :2

Cooking Time :5minutes

INGREDIENTS:

1/4 cup coconut flour

1 tsp. stevia

1 tbsp. ground flaxseed

1/4 tsp baking powder

1/2 cup almond milk

1/4 tsp vanilla extract

1/2 cup low carb vegan cheese

DIRECTIONS:

1. Mix flaxseed in warm water and set aside.
2. Add in the remaining ingredients.
3. Switch on waffle iron and grease with cooking spray.
4. Pour the batter in the waffle machine and cover.
5. Cook the chaffles for about 3-4 minute suites.
6. Once cooked, remove from the waffle machine.
7. Serve with berries and enjoy!

NUTRITION:

Protein: 32% Fat: 63% Carbohydrates: 5%

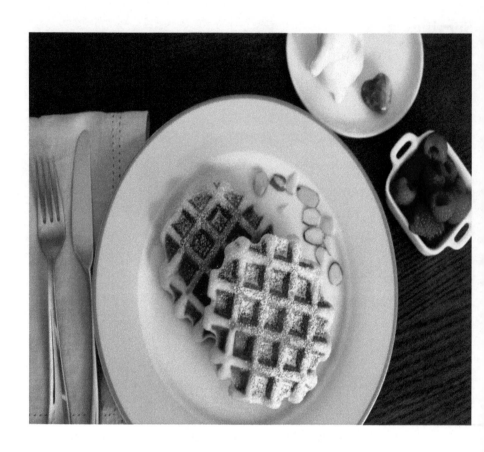

Vegan Chocolate Chaffles

Servings :2

Cooking Time :5minutes

INGREDIENTS:

1/2 cup coconut flour

3 tbsps. cocoa powder

2 tbsps. whole psyllium husk

1/2 teaspoon baking powder

pinch of salt

1/2 cup vegan cheese, softened

1/4 cup coconut milk

DIRECTIONS:

1. Prepare your waffle iron.
2. Mix coconut flour, cocoa powder, baking powder, salt and husk in a bowl and set aside.
3. Add melted cheese and milk and mix well. Let it stand for a few minutes before cooking.
4. Pour batter in the waffle machine and cook for about 3-minute suites.
5. Once chaffles are cooked, carefully remove them from the waffle machine.
6. Serve with vegan ice cream and enjoy!

NUTRITION:

Protein: 42kcal Fat: 82kcal Carbohydrates: 6kcal

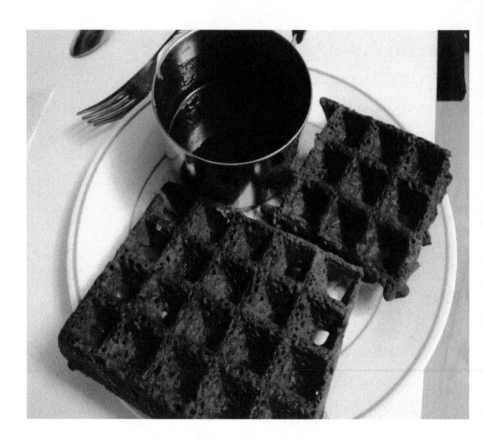

Vegan Waffles With Flaxseed

Servings :2

Cooking Time :5minutes

INGREDIENTS:

1 tbsp. flaxseed meal

2 tbsps. warm water

¼ cup low carb vegan cheese

¼ cup chopped minutest

pinch of salt

2 oz. blueberries chunks

DIRECTIONS:

1. Preheat waffle maker to medium-high heat and grease with cooking spray.
2. Mix flaxseed meal and warm water and set aside to be thickened.
3. After 5 minutes utes' mix together all ingredients in a flax egg.
4. Introduce vegan waffle batter into the center of the waffle iron.
5. Cover and cook for 3-minutes
6. Once cooked, remove the vegan chaffle from the waffle maker and serve.

NUTRITION:

Protein: 42kcal Fat: 82kcal Carbohydrates: 6kcal

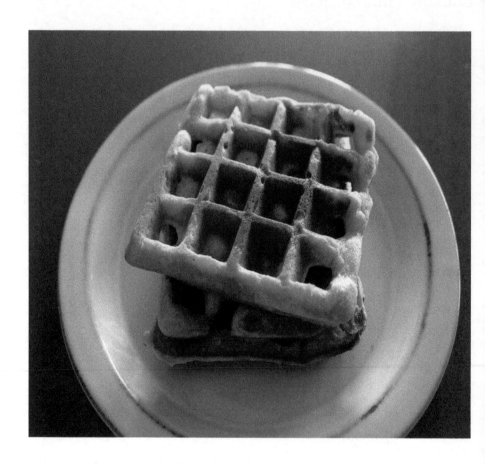

Asparagus Chaffle

Servings :4

Cooking Time :15 Minutes

INGREDIENTS:

Batter

4 eggs

1½ cups grated mozzarella cheese

½ cup grated parmesan cheese

1 cup boiled asparagus, chopped

Salt and pepper to taste

¼ cup almond flour

2 teaspoons baking powder

Other

2 tablespoons cooking spray to brush the waffle maker

¼ cup Greek yogurt for serving

¼ cup chopped almonds for serving

DIRECTIONS:

1. Preheat the waffle maker.
2. Add the eggs, grated mozzarella, grated parmesan, asparagus, salt and pepper, almond flour and baking powder to a bowl.
3. Mix with a fork.

4. Brush the heated waffle maker with cooking spray and add a few tablespoons of the batter.

5. Cover and cook for about 7 minutes depending on your waffle maker.

6. Serve each chaffle with Greek yogurt and chopped almonds.

NUTRITION:

Calories 316, fat 24.9g, carbs 3g, sugar 1.2g, Protein 18.2g, sodium 261mg

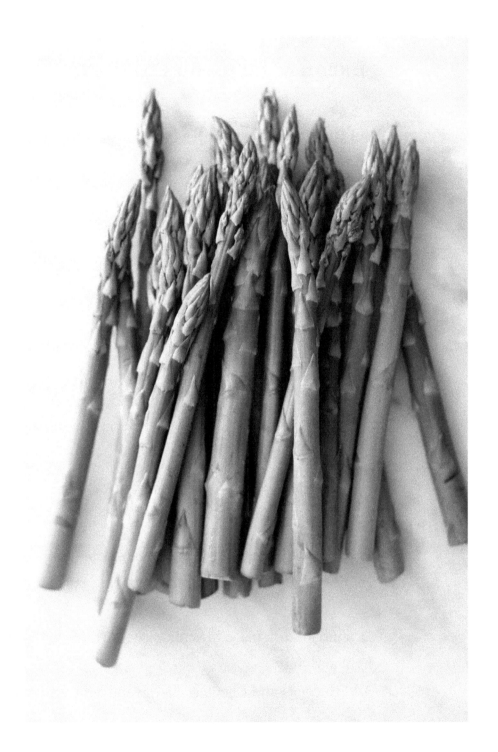

Bacon & Jalapeño Chaffles

Preparation time : 10 minutes

Cooking Time : 15 Minutes

Servings : 2

INGREDIENTS :

      3 tablespoons coconut flour

      1 teaspoon organic baking powder

      ¼ teaspoon salt

      ½ cup cream cheese, softened

      3 large organic eggs

      1 cup sharp Cheddar cheese, shredded

      1 jalapeño pepper, seeded and chopped

      3 cooked bacon slices, crumbled

DIRECTIONS :

1. Preheat a mini waffle iron and then grease it.
2. In a small bowl, place the flour, baking powder and salt and mix well.
3. In a large bowl, place the cream cheese and beat until light and fluffy.
4. Add the eggs and Cheddar cheese and beat until well combined.

5. Add the flour mixture and beat until combined.

6. Fold in the jalapeño pepper.

7. Divide the mixture into 5 portions.

8. Place 1 portion of the mixture into preheated waffle iron and cook for about 5 minutes or until golden brown.

9. Repeat with the remaining mixture.

10. Serve warm with the topping of bacon pieces.

NUTRITION :

Calories: 249Net Carb: 2.9gFat: 20.3gSaturated Fat: 5gCarbohydrates: 4.8gDietary Fiber: 1.9g Sugar: 0.5gProtein: 12.7g

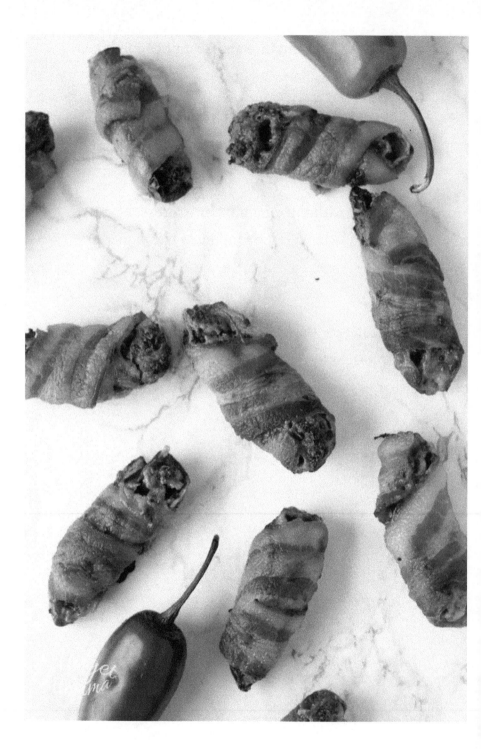

Cheese Broccoli Chaffles

Preparation time : 10 minutes

Cooking Time : 16 Minutes

Servings : 2

INGREDIENTS :

    ½ cup cooked broccoli, chopped finely

    2 organic eggs, beaten

    ½ cup Cheddar cheese, shredded

    ½ cup Mozzarella cheese, shredded

    2 tablespoons Parmesan cheese, grated

    ½ teaspoon onion powder

DIRECTIONS :

1. Preheat a waffle iron and then grease it.
2. Introduce to a medium bowl, all ingredients and mix until well combined.
3. Put half of the mixture in the preheated waffle iron and cook until golden brown, or around 4 minutes.
4. Repeat with the mixture that remains.
5. Serve it hot.

NUTRITION :

Calories: 112Net Carb: 1.2gFat: 8.1gSaturated Fat: 4.3gCarbohydrates: 1.5gDietary Fiber: 0.3g Sugar: 0.5gProtein: 8.

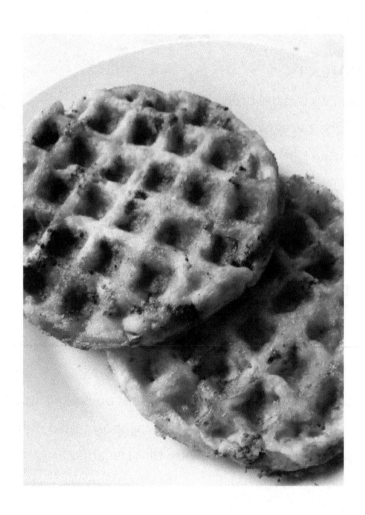

Bacon and Ham Waffle Sandwich

Preparation time : 6 minutes

Cooking Time : 5 Minutes

Servings : 2

INGREDIENTS :

    3 egg

    ½ cup grated Cheddar cheese

    1 Tbsp almond flour

    ½ tsp baking powder

    For the toppings:

    4 strips cooked bacon

    2 pieces Bibb lettuce

    2 slices preferable ham

    2 slices tomato

DIRECTIONS :

1. Turn on the waffle maker to heat and oil it with cooking spray.
2. Combine all chaffle components in a small bowl.
3. Add around ¼ of total batter to the waffle maker and spread to fill the edges. Close and cook for 4 minutes.
4. Remove and let it cool on a rack.
5. Repeat for the second chaffle.

6. Top one chaffle with a tomato slice, a piece of lettuce, and bacon strips, then cover it with a second chaffle.
7. Plate and enjoy.

NUTRITION :

Carbs: 5 g;Fat: 60 g;Protein: 31 g;Calories: 631

Burger Chaffle

Preparation time : 5 minutes

Cooking Time : 10 Minutes

Servings : 2

INGREDIENTS :

For the Cheeseburgers:

1/3 lb beef, ground

½ tsp garlic salt

3 slices American cheese

For the Chaffles:

1 large egg

½ cup mozzarella, finely shredded

Salt and ground pepper to taste

For the Big Mac Sauce:

2 tsp mayonnaise

1 tsp ketchup

To Assemble:

2 tbsp lettuce, shredded

4 dill pickles

2 tsp onion, minced

To assemble burgers:

DIRECTIONS :

1. Take your burger patties and place them on one chaffle. Top with shredded lettuce, onions and pickles.
2. Spread the sauce over the other chaffle and place it on top of the veggies, sauce side down.
3. Enjoy.

NUTRITION :

Calories per **Servings** : 850 Kcal ; Fats: 56 g ; Carbs: 8 g ; Protein: 67 g

Bbq Chicken keto Chaffles

Preparation time : 6 minutes

Cooking Time : 8 Minutes

Servings : 2

INGREDIENTS :

      1 1/3 cups grass-fed cooked chicken, chopped

      ½ cup Cheddar cheese, shredded

      1 tablespoon sugar-free BBQ sauce

      1 organic egg, beaten

      1 tablespoon almond flour

DIRECTIONS :

1. Preheat a mini waffle iron and then grease it.
2. Introduce to a medium bowl, all ingredients and mix until well combined.
3. Put half of the mixture in the preheated waffle iron and cook until golden brown, or around 4 minutes.
4. Repeat with the mixture that remains.
5. Serve it hot.

NUTRITION :

Calories: 320Net Carb: 3.Fat: 16.3gSaturated Fat: 7.6gCarbohydrates: 4gDietary Fiber: 0.4g Sugar: 2gProtein: 36.9g

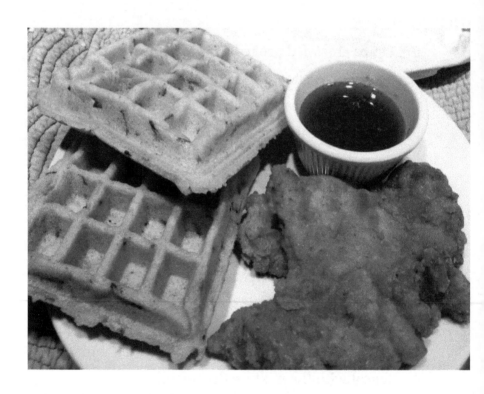

Avocado Chaffle

Preparation time : 6 minutes

Cooking Time : 10 Minutes

Servings : 2

INGREDIENTS :

    ½ avocado, sliced

    ½ tsp lemon juice

    ⅛ tsp salt

    ⅛ tsp black pepper

    1 egg

    ½ cup shredded cheese

    ¼ crumbled feta cheese

    1 cherry tomato, halved

DIRECTIONS :

1. Mash together avocado, lemon juice, salt, and pepper until well-combined.
2. Turn on the waffle maker to heat and oil it with cooking spray.
3. Beat egg in a small mixing bowl.
4. Place ⅛ cup of cheese on the waffle maker, then spread half of the egg mixture over it and top with ⅛ cup of cheese.

5. Close and cook for 3-4 minutes. Repeat for remaining batter.

6. Let chaffles cool for 3-4 minutes, then spread avocado mix on top of each.

7. Top with crumbled feta and cherry tomato halves.

NUTRITION :

Carbs: 5 g;Fat: 19 g;Protein: 7 g;Calories: 232

Zucchini & Onion Chaffles

Preparation time : 10 minutes

Cooking Time : 16 Minutes

Servings : 2

INGREDIENTS :

    2 cups zucchini, grated and squeezed

    ½ cup onion, grated and squeezed

    2 organic eggs

    ½ cup Mozzarella cheese, shredded

    ½ cup Parmesan cheese, grated

DIRECTIONS :

1. Preheat a waffle iron and then grease it.
2. Introduce to a medium bowl, all ingredients and mix until well combined
3. Place ¼ of the mixture into preheated waffle iron and cook for about 4 minutes or until golden brown.
4. Repeat with the remaining mixture.
5. Serve warm.

NUTRITION :

Calories: 92Net Carb: 2.Fat: 5.3gSaturated Fat: 2.3gCarbohydrates: 3.5gDietary Fiber: 0.9g Sugar: 1.8gProtein: 8.6g

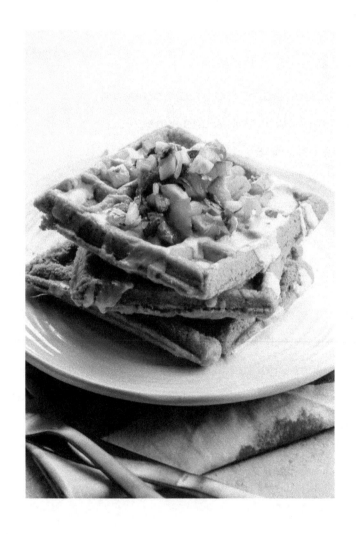

Jalapeño Chaffles

Preparation time : 6 minutes

Cooking Time : 10 Minutes

Servings : 2

INGREDIENTS :

    1 organic egg, beaten

    ½ cup Cheddar cheese, shredded

    ½ tablespoon jalapeño pepper, chopped

    Salt, to taste

DIRECTIONS :

1. Preheat a mini waffle iron and then grease it.
2. Introduce to a medium bowl, all ingredients and mix until well combined.
3. Put a portion of the mixture into preheated waffle iron and cook for about 5 minutes or until golden brown.
4. Repeat with the remaining mixture.
5. Serve warm.

NUTRITION :

Calories: 14et Carb: 0.6gFat: 11.6gSaturated Fat: 6.6gCarbohydrates: 0.6gDietary Fiber: 0g Sugar: 0.4gProtein: 9.8g

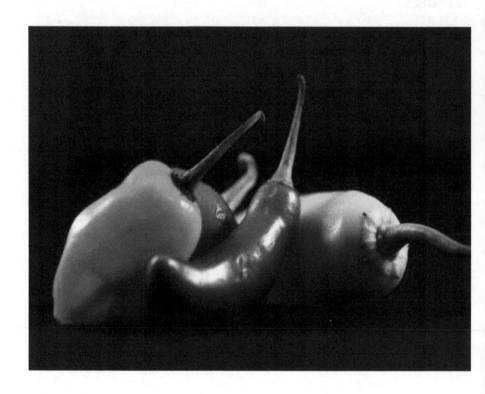

3-cheeses Herbed Chaffles

Preparation time : 10 minutes

Cooking Time : 12 Minutes

Servings : 2

INGREDIENTS :

    4 tablespoons almond flour

    1 tablespoon coconut flour

    1 teaspoon mixed dried herbs

    ½ teaspoon organic baking powder

    ¼ teaspoon garlic powder

    ¼ teaspoon onion powder

    Salt

    freshly ground black pepper

    ¼ cup cream cheese, softened

    3 large organic eggs

    ½ cup Cheddar cheese, grated

    1/3 cup Parmesan cheese, grated

DIRECTIONS :

1. Preheat a waffle iron and then grease it.
2. In a bowl, mix the flours, dried herbs, baking powder and seasoning and mix well.

3. In a separate bowl, put cream cheese and eggs and beat until well combined.

4. Add the flour mixture, cheddar and Parmesan cheese and mix until well combined.

5. Place the desired amount of the mixture into preheated waffle iron and cook for about 2-3 minutes or until golden brown.

6. Repeat with the remaining mixture.

7. Serve warm.

NUTRITION :

Calories: 240Net Carb: 2.6gFat: 19gSaturated Fat: 5gCarbohydrates: 4gDietary Fiber: 1.6g Sugar: 0.7gProtein: 12.3g

Bagel Seasoning Chaffles

Preparation time : 10 minutes

Cooking Time : 20 Minutes

Servings : 2

INGREDIENTS :

    1 large organic egg

    1 cup Mozzarella cheese, shredded

    1 tablespoon almond flour

    1 teaspoon organic baking powder

    2 teaspoons bagel seasoning

    ¼ teaspoon garlic powder

    ¼ teaspoon onion powder

DIRECTIONS :

1. Preheat a mini waffle iron and then grease it.
2. Introduce to a medium bowl, all ingredients and mix until well combined.
3. Place ¼ of the mixture into preheated waffle iron and cook for about 4 minutes or until golden brown.
4. Repeat with the remaining mixture.
5. Serve warm.

NUTRITION :

Calories: 73Net Carb: 2gFat: 5.5gSaturated Fat: 1.5gCarbohydrates: 2.3gDietary Fiber: 0.3g Sugar: 0.9gProtein: 3.7g

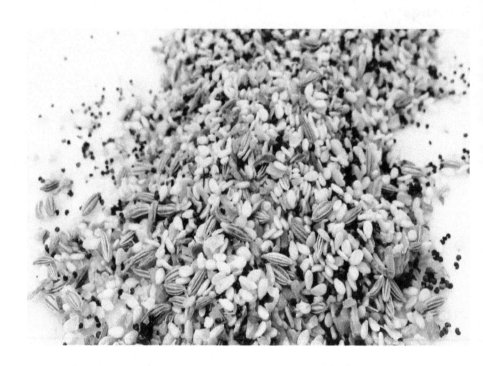

Simple Grilled Cheese Chaffle

Preparation time : 5 minutes

Cooking Time : 10 Minutes

Servings : 2

INGREDIENTS :

      1 large egg

      ½ cup mozzarella cheese

      2 slices yellow American cheese

      2-3 slices cooked bacon, cut in half

      1 tsp butter

      ½ tsp baking powder

DIRECTIONS :

1. Turn on the waffle maker to heat and oil it with cooking spray.
2. Beat egg in a bowl.
3. Add mozzarella, and baking powder.
4. Introduce half of the mix into the waffle maker and cook for minutes.
5. Remove and repeat to make the second chaffle.
6. Layer bacon and cheese slices in between two chaffles.

7. Melt butter in a skillet and add chaffle sandwich to the pan. Fry on each side for 2-3 minutes covered, until cheese has melted.
8. Slice into two on a plate and serve.

NUTRITION :

Carbs: 4 g;Fat: 18 g;Protein: 7 g;Calories: 233

Bbq Rub Chaffles

Preparation time : 10 minutes

Cooking Time : 20 Minutes

Servings : 2

INGREDIENTS :

    2 organic eggs, beaten

    1 cup Cheddar cheese, shredded

    ½ teaspoon BBQ rub

    ¼ teaspoon organic baking powder

DIRECTIONS :

1. Preheat a mini waffle iron and then grease it.
2. Introduce to a medium bowl, all ingredients and mix until well combined.
3. Place ¼ of the mixture into preheated waffle iron and cook for about 5 minutes or until golden brown.
4. Repeat with the remaining mixture.
5. Serve warm.

NUTRITION :

Calories: 14et Carb: 0.7gFat: 11.6gSaturated Fat: 6.6gCarbohydrates: 0.7gDietary Fiber: 0g Sugar: 0.3gProtein: 9.8g

Ham Chaffles

Preparation time : 10 minutes

Cooking Time : 16 Minutes

Servings : 2

INGREDIENTS :

> 2 large organic eggs (yolks and whites separated)
>
> 6 tablespoons butter, melted
>
> 2 scoops unflavored whey protein powder
>
> 1 teaspoon organic baking powder
>
> Salt, to taste
>
> 1 ounce sugar-free ham, chopped finely
>
> 1 ounce Cheddar cheese, shredded
>
> 1/8 teaspoon paprika

DIRECTIONS :

1. Preheat a waffle iron and then grease it.
2. In a bowl place egg yolks, butter, protein powder, baking powder and salt and beat until well combined.
3. Add the ham steak pieces, cheese and paprika and stir to combine.
4. Place 2 egg whites and a pinch of salt in another bowl and with an electric hand mixer and beat until stiff peaks form.

5. Gently wrap the whipped egg albumen into the egg yolk mixture in 2 batches.
6. Place ¼ of the mixture into preheated waffle iron and cook for about 3-4 minutes or until golden brown.
7. Repeat with the remaining mixture.
8. Serve warm.

NUTRITION :

Calories: 288Net Carb: 1.5gFat: 22.8gSaturated Fat: 13.4gCarbohydrates: 1.7gDietary Fiber: 0.2g Sugar: 0.3gProtein: 20.3g

Cheddar Jalapeño Chaffle

Preparation time : 6 minutes

Cooking Time : 5 Minutes

Servings : 2

INGREDIENTS :

    2 large eggs

    ½ cup shredded mozzarella

    ¼ cup almond flour

    ½ tsp baking powder

    ¼ cup shredded cheddar cheese

    2 Tbsp diced jalapeños jarred or canned

    For the toppings:

    ½ cooked bacon, chopped

    2 Tbsp cream cheese

    ¼ jalapeño slices

DIRECTIONS :

1. Turn on the waffle maker to heat and oil it with cooking spray.
2. Mix mozzarella, eggs, baking powder, almond flour, and garlic powder in a bowl.
3. Sprinkle 2 Tbsp cheddar cheese in a thin layer on waffle maker, and ½ jalapeño.

4. Scoop half of the egg mixture on top of the cheese and jalapeños.
5. Cook for minutes, or until done.
6. Repeat for the second chaffle.
7. Top with cream cheese, bacon, and jalapeño slices.

NUTRITION :

Carbs: 5 g;Fat: 1g;Protein: 18 g;Calories: 307

Taco Chaffles

Preparation time : 10 minutes

Cooking Time : 20 Minutes

Servings : 2

INGREDIENTS :

    1 tablespoon almond flour

    1 cup taco blend cheese

    2 organic eggs

    ¼ teaspoon taco seasoning

DIRECTIONS :

1. Preheat a mini waffle iron and then grease it.
2. Introduce to a medium bowl, all ingredients and mix until well combined.
3. Place ¼ of the mixture into preheated waffle iron and cook for about 4 minutes or until golden brown.
4. Repeat with the remaining mixture.
5. Serve warm.

NUTRITION :

Calories: 71Net Carb: 0.7gFat: 5.4gSaturated Fat: 2.2gCarbohydrates: 0.9gDietary Fiber: 0.2g Sugar: 0.3gProtein: 4.5g

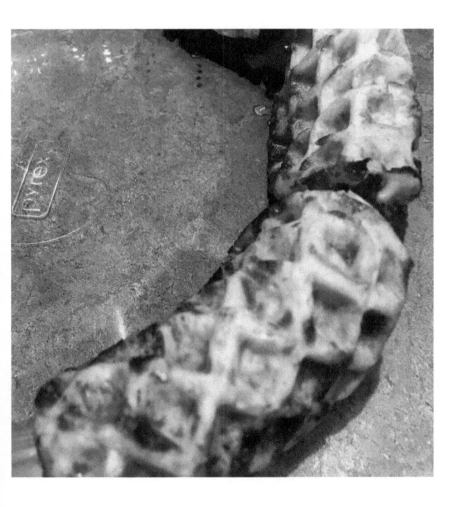

Spinach & Cauliflower Chaffles

Preparation time : 6 minutes

Cooking Time : 10 Minutes

Servings : 2

INGREDIENTS :

½ cup frozen chopped spinach, thawed and squeezed

½ cup cauliflower, chopped finely

½ cup Cheddar cheese, shredded

½ cup Mozzarella cheese, shredded

1/3 cup Parmesan cheese, , shredded

2 organic eggs

1 tablespoon butter, melted

1 teaspoon garlic powder

1 teaspoon onion powder

Salt

freshly ground black pepper

DIRECTIONS :

1. Preheat a waffle iron and then grease it.

2. Introduce to a medium bowl, all ingredients and mix until well combined.

3. Put a portion of the mixture into preheated waffle iron and cook for about 4-5 minutes or until golden brown.
4. Repeat with the remaining mixture.
5. Serve warm.

NUTRITION :

Calories: 320Net Carb: 4gFat: 24.5gSaturated Fat: 14gCarbohydrates: 5gDietary Fiber: 1g Sugar: 1.9gProtein: 20.8g

Rosemary Chaffles

Preparation time : 6 minutes

Cooking Time : 8 Minutes

Servings : 2

INGREDIENTS :

　　1 organic egg, beaten

　　½ cup Cheddar cheese, shredded

　　1 tablespoon almond flour

　　1 tablespoon fresh rosemary, chopped

　　Pinch of salt

　　freshly ground black pepper

DIRECTIONS :

1. Preheat a mini waffle iron and then grease it.
2. For chaffles: In a medium bowl, place all ingredients and with a fork, mix thoroughly.
3. Cook half of the mixture in the preheated waffle iron for about 4 minutes or until golden brown.
4. Repeat with the remaining mixture.
5. Serve warm.

NUTRITION :

Calories: 173Net Carb: 1.1gFat: 13.7gSaturated Fat: 9gCarbohydrates: 2.2gDietary Fiber: 1.1g Sugar: 0.4gProtein: 9.9g

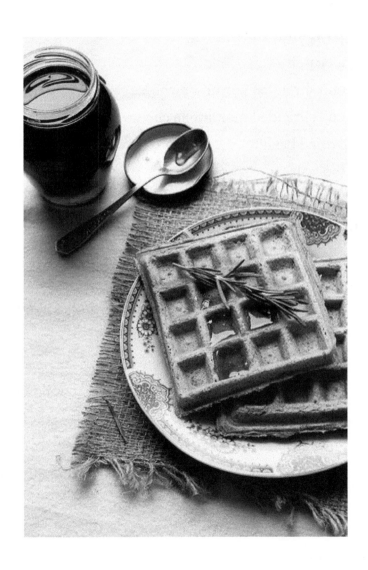

Zucchini Waffles With Peanut Butter

Servings :2

Cooking Time : 5 Minutes

INGREDIENTS :

 1 cup zucchini grated

 1 egg beaten

 1/2 cup shredded parmesan cheese

 1/4 cup shredded mozzarella cheese

 1 tsp dried basil

 1/2 tsp. salt

 1/2 tsp. black pepper

 2 tbsps. peanut butter for topping

DIRECTIONS :

1. Sprinkle salt over zucchini and let it sit for minutes Utes.

2. Squeeze out water from zucchini.

3. Beat egg with zucchini, basil. salt mozzarella cheese, and pepper.

4. Sprinkle ½ of the parmesan cheese over the preheated waffle maker and pour zucchini batter over it.

5. Sprinkle the remaining cheese over it.

6. Cover.

7. Cook zucchini chaffles for about 4-8 minutes.

8. Remove chaffles from the maker and repeat with the remaining batter.

9. Serve with peanut butter on top and enjoy!

NUTRITION :

Protein: 88kcal Fat: 69kcal Carbohydrates: 12kcal

Zucchini Chaffles

Preparation time : 10 minutes

Cooking Time : 18 Minutes

Servings : 2

INGREDIENTS :

    2 large zucchinis, grated and squeezed

    2 large organic eggs

    2/3 cup Cheddar cheese, shredded

    2 tablespoons coconut flour

    ½ teaspoon garlic powder

    ½ teaspoon red pepper flakes, crushed

    Salt, to taste

DIRECTIONS :

1. Preheat a waffle iron and then grease it.
2. Introduce to a medium bowl, all ingredients and mix until well combined.
3. Place ¼ of the mixture into preheated waffle iron and cook for about 4-4½ minutes or until golden brown.
4. Repeat with the remaining mixture.
5. Serve warm.

NUTRITION :

Calories: 159Net Carb: 4.3gFat: 10gSaturated Fat: 5.8gCarbohydrates: 8gDietary Fiber: 3.7g Sugar: 2.Protein: 10.1g

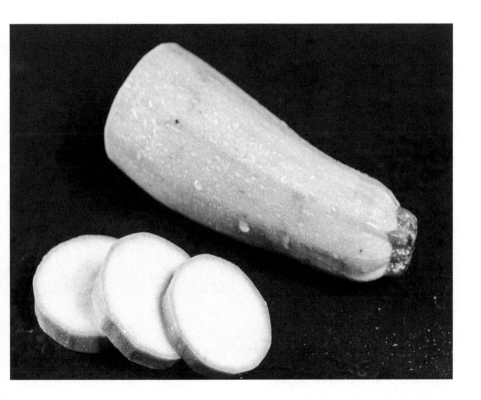

Chicken & Jalapeño Waffles

Preparation time : 6 minutes

Cooking Time : 10 Minutes

Servings : 2

INGREDIENTS :

½ cup grass-fed cooked chicken, chopped

1 organic egg, beaten

¼ cup Cheddar cheese, shredded

2 tablespoons Parmesan cheese, shredded

1 teaspoon cream cheese, softened

1 small jalapeño pepper, chopped

1/8 teaspoon onion powder

1/8 teaspoon garlic powder

DIRECTIONS :

1. Preheat a mini waffle iron and then grease it.
2. Introduce to a medium bowl, all ingredients and mix until well combined.
3. Put a portion of the mixture into preheated waffle iron and cook for about 4-5 minutes or until golden brown.
4. Repeat with the remaining mixture.
5. Serve warm.

NUTRITION :

Calories: 170Net Carb: 0.9gFat: 9.9gSaturated Fat: 5.2gCarbohydrates: 0.1gDietary Fiber: 2. Sugar: 0.5gProtein: 8.6g

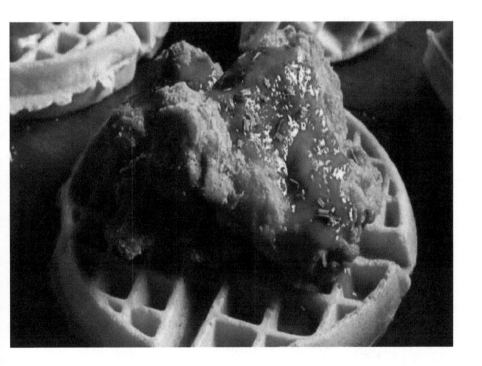

Cauliflower & Chives Chaffles

Servings : 8

Cooking Time : 48 Minutes

INGREDIENTS :

1½ cups cauliflower, grated

½ cup Cheddar cheese, shredded

½ cup Mozzarella cheese, shredded

¼ cup Parmesan cheese, shredded

3 large organic eggs, beaten

3 tablespoons fresh chives, chopped

¼ teaspoon red pepper flakes, crushed

Salt

freshly ground black pepper

DIRECTIONS :

1. Preheat a mini waffle iron and then grease it.
2. In a food processor, Place all the ingredients and pulse until well combined.
3. Divide the mixture into 8 portions.
4. Place 1 portion of the mixture into preheated waffle iron and cook for about 5-6 minutes or until golden brown.
5. Repeat with the remaining mixture.
6. Serve warm.

NUTRITION :

Calories: 10et Carb: 1.2gFat: 7.3gSaturated Fat: 4gCarbohydrates: 1.7gDietary Fiber: 0.5g Sugar: 0.7gProtein: 8.8g

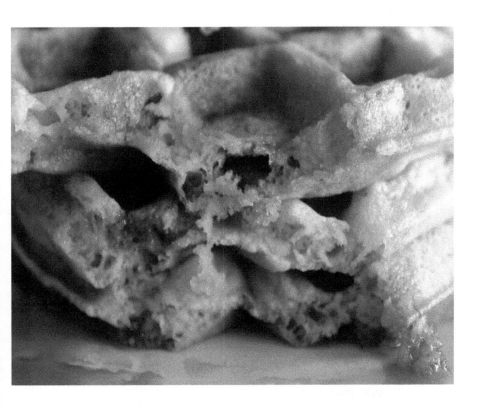

Taco Chaffle Shell

Preparation time : 5 minutes

Cooking Time : 8 Minutes

Servings : 2

INGREDIENTS :

   1 egg white

   ¼ cup shredded Monterey jack cheese

   ¼ cup shredded sharp cheddar cheese

   ¾ tsp water

   1 tsp coconut flour

   ¼ tsp baking powder

   ⅛ tsp chili powder

   Pinch of salt

DIRECTIONS :

1. Turn on the waffle maker to heat and oil it with cooking spray.

2. Mix all components in a bowl.

3. Put half of the batter on the waffle maker and cook for 4 minutes.

4. Remove chaffle and set aside. Repeat for remaining chaffle batter.

5. Turn over a muffin pan and set chaffle between the cups to form a shell. Allow to set for 2-4 minutes.

6. Remove and serve with your favorite taco recipe.

NUTRITION :

Carbs: 4 g;Fat: 19 g;Protein: 18 g;Calories: 258

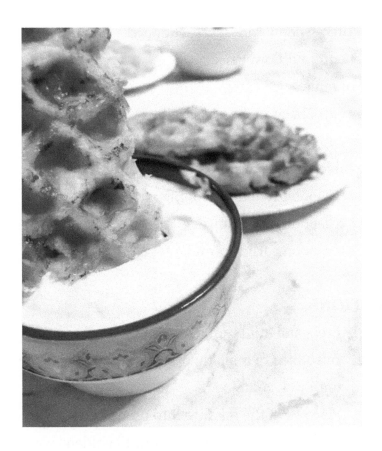

Pepperoni & Cauliflower Chaffles

Preparation time : 10 minutes

Cooking Time : 16 Minutes

Servings : 2

INGREDIENTS :

6 turkey pepperoni slices, chopped

¼ cup cauliflower rice

1 organic egg, beaten

¼ cup Cheddar cheese, shredded

¼ cup Mozzarella cheese, shredded

2 tablespoons Parmesan cheese, grated

½ teaspoon Italian seasoning

¼ teaspoon onion powder

¼ teaspoon garlic powder

DIRECTIONS :

1. Preheat a mini waffle iron and then grease it.
2. Introduce to a medium bowl, all ingredients and mix until well combined.
3. Place ¼ of the mixture into preheated waffle iron and cook for about 4 minutes or until golden brown.
4. Repeat with the remaining mixture.
5. Serve warm.

NUTRITION :

Calories: 103Net Carb: 0.4gFat: 8gSaturated Fat: 3.2gCarbohydrates: 0.8gDietary Fiber: 0.2g Sugar: 0.4gProtein: 10.2g

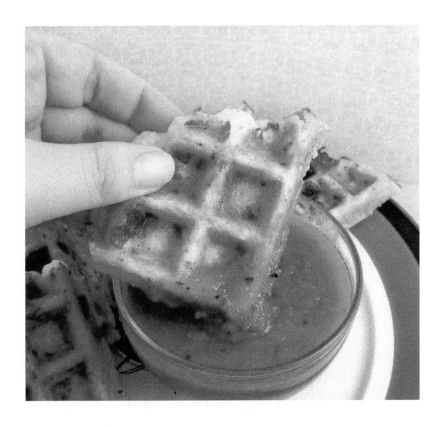

Pulled Pork Chaffle

Servings : 8

Cooking Time : 8 Hours.

INGREDIENTS :

- 1 cup shredded cheddar cheese
- 2 eggs
- ½ tsp BBQ Rub
- 5 lbs pork butt
- ¼ cup BBQ Rub
- 2 Tbsp yellow mustard
- ½ cup sweet BBQ Sauce

DIRECTIONS :

1. Brush mustard on each side of pork butt and season with rub.
2. Set smoker to 0°F. Smoke, uncovered, for about 4 hours, then wrap tightly, using butcher paper, and cook until internal temperature is 205°F.
3. Let pork rest for at least 1 hour before shredding it.
4. Mix cheese and eggs in a small bowl.
5. Scoop out ¼ cup of the mixture and pour into the waffle maker. Cook for minutes.
6. Top chaffles with shredded pork and BBQ sauce.

NUTRITION :

Carbs: 5 g;Fat: 14 g;Protein: 36 g;Calories: 2

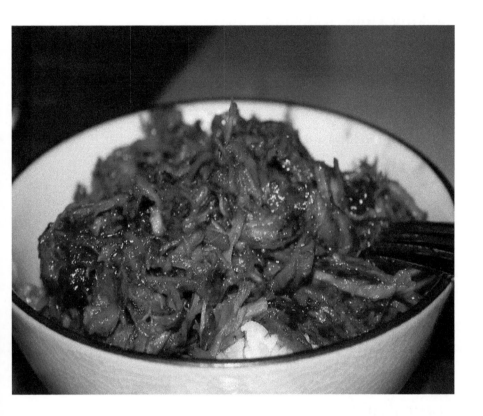

Buffalo Chicken Chaffles

Preparation time : 10 minutes

Cooking Time : 5 Minutes

Servings : 2

INGREDIENTS :

¼ cup almond flour

1 tsp baking powder

2 large eggs

½ cup chicken, shredded

¾ cup sharp cheddar cheese, shredded

¼ cup mozzarella cheese, shredded

¼ cup Red-Hot Sauce + 1 Tbsp for topping

¼ cup feta cheese, crumbled

¼ cup celery, diced

DIRECTIONS :

1. Whisk baking powder and almond flour in a small bowl and set aside.

2. Turn on the waffle maker to heat and oil it with cooking spray.

3. Beat eggs in a large bowl until frothy.

4. Add hot sauce and beat until combined.

5. Mix in flour mixture.

6. Add cheeses and mix until well combined.

7. Fold in chicken.

8. Pour batter into the waffle maker and cook for 4 minutes.

9. Remove and repeat until all batter is used up.

10. Top with celery, feta, and hot sauce.

NUTRITION :

Carbs: 4 g;Fat: 26 g;Protein: 22 g;Calories: 337

Japanese Breakfast Chaffle

Preparation time : 6 minutes

Cooking Time : 10 Minutes

Servings : 2

INGREDIENTS :

    1 egg

    ½ cup shredded mozzarella cheese

    1 Tbsp kewpie mayo

    1 stalk of green onion, chopped

    1 slice bacon, chopped

DIRECTIONS :

1. Turn on the waffle maker to heat and oil it with cooking spray.
2. Beat egg in a small bowl.
3. Add 1 Tbsp mayo, bacon, and ½ green onion. Mix well.
4. Place ⅛ cup of cheese on the waffle maker, then spread half of the egg mixture over it and top with ⅛ cup cheese.
5. Close and cook for 3-4 minutes.
6. Repeat for remaining batter.

7. Transfer to a plate and sprinkle with remaining green onion.

NUTRITION :

Carbs: 1 g;Fat: 16 g;Protein: g;Calories: 183

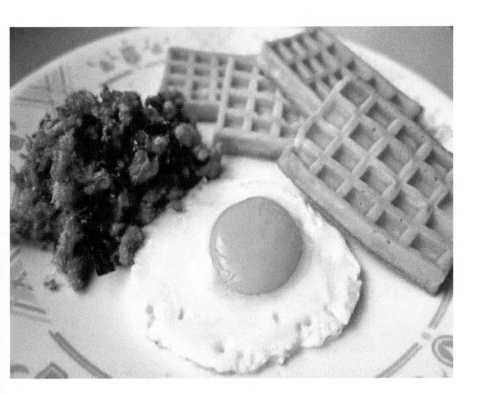

Garlic and Spinach Chaffles

Servings :2

Cooking Time :5minutes

INGREDIENTS :

    1 cup egg whites

    1 tsp. Italian spice

    2 tsps. coconut flour

    ½ tsp. Vanilla

    1 tsp. baking powder

    1 tsp. baking soda

    1 cup mozzarella cheese, grated

    1/2 tsp. garlic powder

    1 cup chopped spinach

DIRECTIONS :

1. Switch on your square waffle maker. Spray with non-stick spray.
2. Beat egg whites with a beater, until fluffy and white.
3. Add pumpkin puree, pumpkin pie spice, coconut flour in egg whites and beat again.
4. Stir in the cheese, powder, garlic powder, baking soda, and powder.
5. Sprinkle chopped spinach on a waffle maker

6. Pour the batter in waffle maker over chopped spinach

7. Close the maker and cook for about 4-5 minutes Utes.

8. Remove chaffles from the maker.

9. Serve hot and enjoy!

NUTRITION :

Protein: 88kcal Fat: 69kcal Carbohydrates: 12kcal

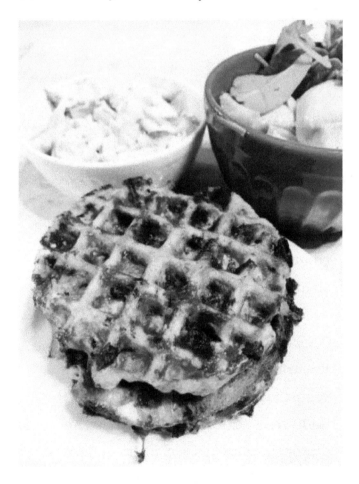

Chaffle Sandwich

Preparation time : 6 minutes

Cooking Time : 8 Minutes

Servings : 2

INGREDIENTS :

> Chaffle bread:
>
> ½ cup mozzarella cheese, shredded
>
> 1 egg
>
> 1 tbsp green onion, diced
>
> ½ tsp Italian seasoning
>
> Sandwich
>
> ½ lb bacon, pre-cooked
>
> 1 small lettuce
>
> 1 medium tomato sliced
>
> 1 tbsp mayo

DIRECTIONS :

1. Preheat your mini waffle maker.
2. Whip the egg in a small mixing bowl.
3. Add the seasonings, cheese, and onion. Mix thoroughly until it's well incorporated.
4. Add a teaspoon of shredded cheese to the waffle maker and cook for 30 seconds.

5. Place half the batter in the waffle pan and cook for 4 minutes.
6. Once the first chaffle is done, repeat the process with the remaining mixture.
7. Once ready remove and place on a plate. Top with the mayo, lettuce, bacon, and tomato.
8. Place the second chaffle on top, slice into 2 and enjoy!

NUTRITION :

Calories per **Preparation tim e** : 6 minutes40 Kcal ; Fats: 18 g ; Carbs: 2 g ; Protein: 17 g

Cauliflower & Italian Seasoning Chaffles

Preparation time : 10 minutes

Cooking Time : 20 Minutes

Servings : 2

INGREDIENTS :

1 cup cauliflower rice

¼ teaspoon garlic powder

½ teaspoon Italian seasoning

Salt

freshly ground black pepper

½ cup Mexican blend cheese, shredded

1 organic egg, beaten

½ cup Parmesan cheese, shredded

DIRECTIONS :

1. Preheat a mini waffle iron and then grease it.
2. In a blender, add all the ingredients except Parmesan cheese and pulse until well combined.
3. Place 1½ tablespoon of the Parmesan cheese in the bottom of preheated waffle iron.
4. Place ¼ of the egg mixture over cheese and sprinkle with the ½ tablespoon of the Parmesan cheese.
5. Cook for about 4-minutes or until golden brown.

6. Repeat with the remaining mixture and Parmesan cheese.
7. Serve warm.

NUTRITION :

Calories: 127Net Carb: 2gFat: 9gSaturated Fat: 5.3gCarbohydrates: 2.7gDietary Fiber: 0.7g Sugar: 1.5gProtein: 9.2g

Breakfast Chaffle

Preparation time : 6 minutes

Cooking Time : 5 Minutes

Servings : 2

INGREDIENTS :

2 eggs

½ cup shredded mozzarella cheese

For the toppings:

2 ham slices

1 fried egg

DIRECTIONS :

1. Mix eggs and cheese in a small bowl.
2. Turn on the waffle maker to heat and oil it with cooking spray.
3. Introduce half of the batter into the waffle maker.
4. Cook for 2-minutes, remove, and repeat with remaining batter.
5. Place egg and ham between two chaffles to make a sandwich.

NUTRITION :

Carbs: 1 g;Fat: 8 g;Protein: 9 g;Calories: 115

Chaffle Cuban Sandwich

Preparation time : 5 minutes

Cooking Time : 10 Minutes

Servings : 2

INGREDIENTS :

　　1 large egg

　　1 Tbsp almond flour

　　1 Tbsp full-fat Greek yogurt

　　⅛ tsp baking powder

　　¼ cup shredded Swiss cheese

　　For the Filling:

　　3 oz roast pork

　　2 oz deli ham

　　1 slice Swiss cheese

　　3-5 sliced pickle chips

　　½ Tbsp Dijon mustard

DIRECTIONS :

1. Turn on the waffle maker to heat and oil it with cooking spray.

2. Beat egg, yogurt, almond flour, and baking powder in a bowl.

3. Sprinkle ¼ Swiss cheese on the hot waffle maker. Top with half of the egg mixture, then add ¼ of the cheese on top. Close and cook for 5 minutes, until golden brown and crispy.
4. Repeat with remaining batter.
5. Layer pork, ham, and cheese slice in a small microwaveable bowl. Microwave for seconds, until cheese melts.
6. Spread the inside of the chaffle with mustard and top with pickles. Invert bowl onto chaffle top so that cheese is touching pickles. Place bottom chaffle onto pork and serve.

NUTRITION :

Carbs: 4 g;Fat: 46 g;Protein: 33 g;Calories: 522

Sausage & Veggie Chaffles

Preparation time : 10 minutes

Cooking Time : 20 Minutes

Servings : 2

INGREDIENTS :

 1/3 cup unsweetened almond milk

 4 medium organic eggs

 2 tablespoons gluten-free breakfast sausage, cut into slices

 2 tablespoons broccoli florets, chopped

 2 tablespoons bell peppers, seeded and chopped

 2 tablespoons mozzarella cheese, shredded

DIRECTIONS :

1. Preheat a waffle iron and then grease it.
2. In a medium bowl, add the almond milk and eggs and beat well.
3. Place the remaining **INGREDIENTS** and stir to combine well.
4. Place desired amount of the mixture into preheated waffle iron.
5. Cook for about minutes.
6. Repeat with the remaining mixture.

106

7. Serve warm.

NUTRITION :

Calories 132 Net Carbs 1.2 g Total Fat 9.2 g Saturated Fat 3.5 gCholesterol 117 mgSodium 216 mg Total Carbs 1.4 gFiber 0.2 g Sugar 0.5 gProtein 11.1 g

Lightning Source UK Ltd.
Milton Keynes UK
UKHW020743250621
386134UK00001B/35